Mogens S

CW00530100

Lithium Treatment of Manic-Depressive Illness

A Practical Guide

5th, revised edition
1 figure and 5 tables, 1993

EASTBOURNE
01/10/03

KARGER

Basel · Freiburg · Paris · London · New York ·
New Delhi · Singapore · Tokyo · Sydney

Mogens Schou

MD, Dr. med., Dr. h.c. mult., FRC Psych. (Hon.) is Emeritus Professor of Biological Psychiatry at Aarhus University and Emeritus Research Director of the Psychopharmacology Research Unit, the Psychiatric Hospital, Risskov (Denmark)

1st edition 1980
2nd, revised edition 1983
3rd edition 1986
4th, revised edition 1989
5th, revised edition 1993

Library of Congress Cataloging-in-Publication Data
Schou, Mogens.
Lithium treatment of manic-depressive illness: a practical guide / Mogens Schou. – 5th. rev. ed.
Rev. ed. of 4th ed. which was an English translation of the Danish:
Lithiumbehandling af manio-depressiv sygdom.
Includes bibliographical references and index.
(alk. paper)
1. Lithium – Therapeutic use. 2. Manic-depressive psychoses – Chemotherapy. I. Title.
[DNLM: 1. Bipolar Disorder – drug therapy – popular works.
2. Lithium – therapeutic use – popular works. WM 207 S376L 1993]
RC483.5.L5S3613 1993
616.89'5061 – dc20

Drug Dosage
The author and publisher have exerted every effort to ensure that drug selection and dosage set forth in this text are in accord with current recommendations and practice at the time of publication. However, in view of ongoing research, changes in government regulations, and the constant flow of information relating to drug therapy and drug reactions, the reader is urged to check the package insert for each drug for any change in indications and dosage and for added warnings and precautions. This is particularly important when the recommended agent is a new and/or infrequently employed drug.

All rights reserved.
No part of this publication may be translated into other languages, eproduced or utilized in any form or by any means, electronic or mechanical, including photocopying, recording, microcopying, or by any information storage and retrieval system, without permission in writing from the publisher.

© Copyright 1993 by S. Karger AG, P.O. Box, CH– 4009 Basel (Switzerland)
Printed in Switzerland on acid-free paper by Thür AG Offsetdruck, Pratteln
ISBN 3–8055–5667–5

Contents

Acknowledgments

I wish to thank the patients, relatives, nurses, general practitioners, and psychiatrists who took the time to read and comment on my manuscript.

Mogens Schou

Preface

to the 5th, Revised Edition

The first edition of this book appeared in 1980 and was received kindly by reviewers and readers. Later editions, including the present one, have been revised in order to bring them up to date.

The revisions have incorporated scientific progress made within recent years, especially the observation that lithium treatment can be carried out with lower doses and blood levels than used formerly. This has not led to any significant lowering of the efficacy but to a marked reduction of the frequency and intensity of side effects.

Reader reactions have also led to revisions of the text. Sections that were difficult to understand or insufficiently informative have been rewritten; other sections found of little interest have been left out. I have tried to include the patients' own experiences of being manic-depressive and in lithium treatment.

Prophylactic lithium treatment, as any other long-term drug therapy, makes demands on both patients and physicians. The patients must follow the rules of the game, and the physicians owe it to their patients to be acquainted with modern treatment guidelines and precautions. Patients and physicians are jointly responsible for using lithium treatment safely and effectively. I hope this book may contribute to their joint satisfaction with good treatment results.

Mogens Schou

1   Introduction

For Whom Is This Book Written?

The book is written for manic-depressive patients receiving treatment with lithium, for their relatives, and for others who may be interested and involved in the subject. It contains information which is important for doctors and nurses, and hopefully it may form the basis for discussions between doctor and patient so that both will become more familiar with this special mood disease and its treatment with lithium.

What Does the Book Deal with?

It deals only a little with manic-depressive illness but much with the treatment of this illness with lithium. Further information about the disease may be found in the list of supplementary reading presented at the end of the book.

Lithium treatment is described in detail, and emphasis is placed on measures that are of importance for its most effective application. It is imperative that patients, relatives, and doctors work closely together if the treatment is to have the optimum effect with a minimum of inconvenience and risk.

What Can the Book Be Used for?

New patients, that is patients who are about to start or who recently started lithium treatment, are told what they can expect in terms of treatment gain and what they can be exposed to in terms of risk and inconvenience. It may also serve to give instructions. Patients with diabetes, for instance, are co-responsible for their diet and their treatment with insulin or tablets. In the same way, manic-depressive patients on lithium must learn about rules they should follow and situations which demand particular attention. For more experienced lithium patients, the book may serve as a reference volume regarding length and effects of treatment.

What the Book Cannot Provide

The book cannot replace the patient's contact with psychiatrist or general practitioner. It is the doctor who makes the diagnosis and institutes the treatment, and no written description of the disease, however thorough, can replace the doctor's experience and assessment. Nor can the book replace treatment control or the doctor's careful instructions to the patient. It is not intended as an independent guide but as an aid in the cooperation between patient and doctor.

On Reading the Book

The book has been written for both new and more experienced patients, for those who want extensive information about lithium as well as for those who are looking for essential instructions. Since readers may have different interests, it is important to note that the various sections of the book can be read in a sequence that differs from that chosen here.

2   Glossary

I have tried to avoid unnecessary medical words but have used a number of technical terms because they give a precise meaning. The words are explained in the list below. The explanations have been phrased so that they are valid in the context in which they are used; general definitions have not been aimed for.

Abstinence Phenomena. Unpleasant signs and symptoms which appear in drug addicts when the drug is suddenly withdrawn.

Acute. Short, active course.

Antidepressants. Drugs for the treatment of depression.

Bipolar. Manic-depressive course with both manias and depressions.

Chronic. Protracted course.

Dehydration. Water deficiency.

Delusion. Wrong idea which cannot be corrected through reasoning or sensory impressions.

Diuretics. 'Water pills', drugs which enhance urine production.

Dummy Tablets (Placebo). Inactive tablets which in appearance are similar to the tablets under investigation but which do not contain the active compound. They are used in controlled treatment trials in order to distinguish between imagined effects and true treatment effects.

Edema. Swelling due to accumulation of fluid in the tissues.

Electric Convulsive Treatment. Treatment through electrical stimulation of the brain; used for the treatment of depression and sometimes of mania.

Episode. Manic or depressive disease attack.

Goiter. Enlargement of the thyroid gland with swelling of the neck.

Hallucination. Sensory illusion, false sensory experience.

Interaction. Effect exerted by one drug on the effect of another drug.

Interval. The period between a manic or depressive episode and the following manic or depressive episode.

Ion. Positively or negatively charged atom or atom group.

mg. Milligram, one thousandth gram.

Mixed State. Disease state with simultaneous symptoms of mania and depression.

mmol. Millimole, chemical quantity; in this book 7 mg of lithium ion.

mmol/l. Millimoles per liter, concentration of a substance; in this book the lithium concentration in blood serum.

Myxedema. Pathological condition with reduced metabolism, caused by lowered function of the thyroid gland.

Neuroleptics. Drugs for the treatment of non-depressive mental illness.

Polydipsia. Increased thirst and intake of fluid.

Polyuria. Increased production of urine with frequent urination.

Prophylaxis. Prevention of disease; in this book used about the prevention of manic and depressive recurrences.

Recurrent. Disease course with repeated attacks.

Relapse. Recurrence of a disease from which the patient has previously suffered; in this book used especially about manic or depressive recurrences.

Salts. Chemical compounds consisting of a positively charged ion, usually a metal ion, and a negatively charged ion, the anion. Lithium carbonate and lithium citrate are salts used for treatment. Ordinary table salt is sodium chloride.

Serum. The clear fluid which separates from the blood corpuscles when the blood has been left for some time to clot.

Serum Creatinine. Creatinine concentration in serum, a measure of kidney function.

Serum Lithium. Lithium concentration in serum, expressed in mmol/l.

Serum TSH. Concentration of thyroid-stimulating hormone in serum, a measure of thyroid gland function.

Slow-Release Tablets. Tablets from which the drug is released slowly in the gastrointestinal tract.

Sodium. Metallic element. The sodium ion, Na^+, occurs widely distributed in the organism and is part of ordinary table salt, sodium chloride.

Teratogenic Effect. Production of malformations in the unborn child.

Therapy. Treatment of disease; in this book used about treatment of the individual manic or depressive episodes.

Tremor. Trembling, especially of the hands.

Unipolar. Manic-depressive course with recurrent depressions only and no manias.

4

3   Manic-Depressive Illness and Its Treatment

Manic-Depressive Illness

Manic-depressive illness occurs in attacks or episodes. These may be attacks of mania, that is periods with abnormal elation and increased activity, or they may be attacks of depression, periods with abnormal sadness and melancholy. The same patients may have both manias and depressions. Some patients have only depressions and a few only manias. Occasionally the disease presents a mixture of manic and depressive features; this is referred to as a mixed state.

Manic-depressive illness is a fairly frequent disease. About 1–2 persons out of every 100 develop, some time in their life, symptoms of such severity that hospital treatment is required. Women fall ill more frequently than men. The disease often starts between 30 and 50 years of age, but it may appear for the first time at 15–20 years (in rare cases even in childhood) and as late as 60–70 years.

Manic and depressive episodes present themselves differently in different persons and in the individual patient from time to time. Characteristic disease features are described in the following, but not all are present during each episode.

Mania

Prominent features of manic episodes are elation, easily aroused anger, and increased mental speed. The elation varies from unusual zest to uninhibited enthusiasm. The anger mostly takes the form of irritability. The patients become annoyed if other people do not immediately follow their many ideas. Intellectual activity takes place with lightning speed, ideas race through the head, speech flows with great rapidity and almost without breaks, puns alternate with caustic repartee.

During a manic episode the patients' evaluation of themselves is changed. They are excessively self-confident and lack self-criticism. This produces a previously unknown vigor, and when that is combined with a wealth of ideas, indefatigability, and lack of inhibitions, the consequences are often unfortunate. During manic episodes the patients may destroy their marriage, spoil their reputation, or ruin themselves financially.

Manic patients usually sleep very little. They rarely feel tired and are kept awake by the rapid flow of ideas. Sexual activity may be increased. The patients often neglect eating and may lose weight. Combination of violent activity, lowered food intake, and too little sleep may lead to physical exhaustion.

Manic patients often fail to realize that they are ill. On the contrary, they feel unusually well and find it difficult to understand that their nearest and dearest are of a different opinion. It may be a serious strain on marriage and family feelings when the relatives consider the patient ill and treatment indicated, and in this situation much love, tact, and tolerance are required from all sides. The situation can become very difficult, and it may be made worse by rejection and indignation from outsiders who fail to understand that illness is involved.

Mania in a mild degree is called hypomania.

Depression

Depressions are in many respects the opposite of manias. They are characterized by sadness, lacking self-confidence, and lowered mental speed. The sadness may vary from a slight feeling of being 'blue' to black despair. Frequently the patients feel painfully that their emotions are 'dried out'; they want to cry but are unable to do so. Weighed down by feelings of guilt and selfreproaches they may consider or commit suicide.

The patients' courage and self-confidence have disappeared. They are resigned, lack initiative and energy, feel that obstacles are insurmountable, and have difficulty making even trivial decisions. Due to the low self-esteem and the feelings of inadequacy the patients often fear being with other people.

The mental speed of depressed patients is usually low. Ideas are few, thoughts move slowly, and memory function is impaired. The patients feel tired and heavy. The condition may, on the other hand, be characterized by overwhelming anxiety; the patients are then agitated and restless.

Sleep disturbances are frequent. Occasionally there is increased need for sleep, but more often the patients have difficulty sleeping. Some patients find it hard to fall asleep, others wake up frequently during the night, and others again may wake up early with feelings of anxiety. There is often variation in the mood over the day. It is low late in the night and in the early morning, everything is black, the desire to stay in bed is overwhelming, and the first hours of the day are difficult to get through.

Depressions are often accompanied by physical changes. The muscles give the impression of being slack, the facial expression is static, and motions are slow. There may be constipation, menstruation may stop, and sexual interest and activity usually decrease. Appetite is reduced with resulting loss of weight.

Cessation of depression is sometimes followed by a light and transient mania, which may be seen as a reaction to the depression or as a sign of relief that it stopped.

Mixed State

In addition to manias and depressions, manic-depressive disease may present mixed states during which there are signs of mania and depression at the same time. The patients may be sad and without energy but also irritable, or they may be manic and restless and yet feel an underlying melancholy. Mixed states may occur as independent episodes, but they are seen more often during transition from mania to depression or from depression to mania. During periods of transition the condition may alternate between mania and depression several times within the same day.

Interval

During the intervals between episodes the patients often enjoy complete mental health. They may, like others, have good and bad periods, but not all mood changes are abnormal.

Course

Manias and depressions and the intervals between them vary considerably in length both from patient to patient and in the individual patient. As a rough approximation it may be estimated that untreated manic and depressive episodes last 3–6 months, but some episodes are shorter and many longer. There are patients with regularly occurring episodes, for example once a year, but they are exceptions.

Manic-depressive illness may take two different courses. They may represent different diseases. Patients with a *unipolar course* suffer repeated depressive episodes but no manias. Patients with a *bipolar course* experience both manias and depressions. The rare cases with only manias are counted as belonging to the bipolar form, because usually these patients sooner or later have depressions.

As a general rule, episodes tend to occur with shorter intervals over the years, but the course shows much individual variation. A few patients experience only one manic or depressive episode, but most patients have more. Repeated disease episodes may ruin an education.

Admission to Hospital

Mild manias and depressions may be treated at home, but even moderately severe episodes should be treated in hospital. Most patients are admitted voluntarily, but compulsory admission may become necessary when the patients lack insight. Under these circumstances the doctor has an obligation to act in what he considers the patient's best interest.

The Nature of the Illness

We do not know what causes the appearance of manic and depressive episodes. Some persons may be genetically predisposed in such a way that they respond more readily than others with mania or depression to internal and external influences. Insufficient resolution of deep personality problems may play a role. It is possible that changes in the metabolism of the brain are of significance for the development of episodes. Both psychological and non-psychological stresses seem able to precipitate episodes, but often it is not possible to find a precipitating factor.

There is presumably a complex interaction between the effects of internal and external influences in persons with varying degrees of vulnerability and resistance, and both psychological and non-psychological (medical) treatment methods are in use. The question is not so much one of choosing between psychological treatment and drug treatment, as how to combine the two treatments profitably. The subject of this book is treatment with a drug, lithium, and the introductory chapters deal primarily with medical treatment methods. But later in the book it will be described how treatment with lithium and psychological treatment of the patients' personal problems may support and supplement each other.

The Diagnosis of Manic-Depressive Illness

In some instances it is easy for the physician to decide that a patient has manic-depressive illness and may profit from treatment with antidepressant drugs or electric convulsive treatment or possibly, if recurrences are frequent, lithium. But in other cases the diagnosis may present difficulties. Persons with predisposition for manic-depressive illness differ in personality and respond individually to the disease episodes, which therefore may differ somewhat in appearance from the typical cases described in textbooks and on the preceding pages. The physician must evaluate not only the symptoms now present but also previous disease episodes, the condition between episodes, the occurrence of mental disease in the family, etc. Sorting and assessment of information may make considerable demands on the physician's experience, perspicacity and intuition. A reliable diagnosis can often be made only by a trained psychiatrist, and even experienced psychiatrists may be in doubt.

The appearance of a clearly manic episode usually establishes the diagnosis; it is much more difficult when depressive features are predominant. Sadness and feelings of unhappiness need not necessarily be signs of the kind of depression ('endogenous' depression) which is part of manic-depressive illness. They may be expressions of an ordinary grief reaction to tragic events, or they may be signs of depression that has arisen as a reaction to severe mental stress ('exogenous' or 'psychogenic' or 'reactive' depression). Depressive symptoms may also appear as part of a neurotic condition or be secondary to senility or develop because the patient suffers from grave physical disease. These forms of depression should not be treated with electric convulsive treatment or antidepressants or lithium, and it is therefore important that the diagnosis is correct. It is a serious matter if a manic-depressive patient's illness is not recognized so that he is deprived of effective drug treatment, for example with lithium. But it is equally serious if lithium treatment is given for years to a person who does not suffer from manic-depressive illness. Not only does this produce unnecessary side effects, but labelling with a diagnosis and allocation of a patient role may in themselves counteract maturation and improvement.

When Are Manic-Depressive Patients Ill?

Patients with manic-depressive illness at times find themselves in a manic or depressive episode and at other times in a healthy interval, and transition from one to the other condition can be very gradual. It is not always easy to decide when manic-depressive patients are ill and when they are healthy. What for one person may be normal behavior will for another be clearly abnormal, and assessment of the condition must be based on knowledge of the person in question. Frequently the patient and family know from previous episodes the signs indicating that an episode is on the way.

Special difficulties are encountered when patients in the early phase of a mania feel healthy and in excellent condition, while family and physician sense that things are getting out of control. Marital relations, family situation, money matters, working conditions and many other psychological and social factors influence the decision whether treatment and possibly hospital admission are necessary.

Are Manic-Depressive Patients in Fact 'Patients'?

In this book I use the term 'patients' about persons who suffer from manic-depressive illness, but I do it reluctantly. The term is appropriate when the persons are in a manic or depressive episode which has necessitated treatment or hospital admission. It is much more dubious when it is used at a time when they are in an interval or about persons with previous manic-depressive attacks who are kept free of episodes through prophylactic lithium treatment. Under these circumstances they are not 'ill', and many of them may prefer to avoid the patient label with its overtones of hospital world and passivity. But I have not been able to find another term which is short and handy. Later in the book it will be described how important it is that persons in lithium treatment replace the passive patient role with active personal effort and responsibility.

On Being Manic-Depressive

Textbooks in psychiatry often stress that manic-depressive patients are completely healthy and entirely free of disease signs during the intervals between manic and depressive episodes, at least if they have the disease in typical form. This is correct, at least in large measure, and accentuation of the matter draws the students' attention to an important difference from certain other mental diseases which in spite of variable intensity are characterized by persisting disease signs. For the manic-depressive patient it may be of value to learn that the manic or depressive episode will pass and that it will pass without leaving permanent changes.

It would, however, be more than strange if patient and family were left entirely unaffected by such violent experiences as manias and depressions. Acts carried out during mania or depression may have had unfortunate consequences. Marital wounds may heal slowly. Patients with frequent episodes have difficulty finding their own identity, because they are seen by themselves and others as different persons when they are manic, when they are depressed, and when they are in an interval. Many people with manic-depressive experiences feel uncertainty about when they are 'normal', when they are too high, and when they are on the way down. Perpetual watching for signs of disease may lead to introspection that is troublesome for the patients themselves and the family.

Patients with severe manic and depressive episodes often become part of a particular social pattern in which spouse, children, friends, and associates each play a role in a combined effort to mitigate the consequences of the incessant mood changes. In protracted cases the family hardly knows an existence that is not dominated by fear of imminent disaster, depressive suicide attempts or manic deeds of misjudgement. The atmosphere becomes one of constant vigilance, plans can only be tentative, and activities are curbed by the necessity of subordinating everything to the whims of the recurrent disease. The relatives are often in need of psychological support, and it is important that the physician keeps them informed about what is happening, including while the patient is hospitalized.

This sombre picture should, however, not obscure the fact that manic-depressive illness also may provide positive experiences. These are associated with the mild manias, which give improved self-confidence, sensitivity, and resolution, increased sexual intensity, renewed inspiration and creative ability, and a wonderful feeling of social ease. During these periods depressive anxiety and fear of depression disappear, and the patients feel they can accept themselves. Depressive episodes are rarely remembered for the good, but occasionally depressions may draw the family closer together, and depressive experiences may increase the understanding of other people in difficulty.

Treatment of Manic-Depressive Illness

Manic-depressive illness may be treated with therapies other than lithium, and often these are preferable. Occasionally they may be combined with lithium. Psychological support and psychotherapy may be of value during the intervals and in patients with mild episodes.

Electric Convulsive Treatment (ECT)

ECT is carried out in the following manner: During narcosis certain parts of the brain are stimulated electrically through electrodes placed on the skin. This elicits a seizure, but since the muscles are relaxed with a drug, the seizure manifests as muscle twitchings only. The patients do not feel the treatment, but during the following hours they may have some headache and feel tenderness of the muscles. Transitory impairment of memory may occur.

ECT may be used to treat mania but is used primarily for severe depressions; treatment 2–4 times a week for 3–4 weeks leads to amelioration of symptoms in most patients. ECT may be given during hospital admission or on an outpatient basis.

Neuroleptics

For treatment of agitation the so-called neuroleptics are often used. They are sedative drugs like, for example, chlorpromazine (Largactil, Thorazine) or haloperidol (Haldol). Neuroleptics exert a powerful tranquillizing effect on anxiety, restlessness, and tension. They also attenuate or relieve hallucinations and delusions. Neuroleptics are not specific for any single disease. They may be used in the treatment of mania, possibly together with lithium, and they may be used in depressions that are accompanied by delusions. Neuroleptics may produce side effects involving the muscles and the nervous system.

Antidepressants

Antidepressants act, as the name indicates, on depression but only on abnormal depression; they are without effect on ordinary sadness or grief. They are drugs like, for example, imipramine (Tofranil) and amitriptyline (Elavil, Tryptizol).

Side effects of antidepressants may include tiredness, dryness of the mouth, tremor, constipation, difficulty in urinating, and a tendency to faint. Changes in heart rate and rhythm may occur, and careful evaluation is necessary in patients with cardiac disease.

Treatment with antidepressants is continued for some time after disappearance of the symptoms, for example 3–4 months. Occasionally this precipitates episodes of mania, and patients with previous attacks of mania may have to discontinue antidepressant treatment earlier. If patients with a bipolar course need prophylactic treatment, they should be given lithium. Patients with a unipolar course may be treated prophylactically with either lithium or antidepressants.

Lithium Treatment of Manic-Depressive Illness

What Is Lithium?

Lithium is a metallic element which was discovered by a Swedish chemist, *August Arfwedson,* in 1818. He gave it the name of lithium, derived from the Greek word lithos, stone, because it was found in a mineral. Lithium has widespread occurrence in nature, for example in small amounts in plant and animal tissues and in the human organism. It is produced from lithium-containing minerals such as spodumene, amblygonite, lepidolite and petalite. Most of the lithium which is used in Western Europe and the Americas is mined in North Carolina, USA. Lithium and lithium compounds have many technical uses: in the ceramic industry, for the production of alloys, as an adjunct to greases, for the production of electric batteries, in aluminium production, for the heat shields of space ships, and in the production of hydrogen bombs.

Only a small fraction of the lithium produced is used for medical purposes. As a drug, lithium is always used in the form of one of its salts, for example lithium carbonate or lithium citrate. It is the lithium part of these salts, the lithium ion, Li^+, which is effective medically, and in principle it is without importance whether one uses one or the other salt.

The History of Lithium Treatment

Before 1949

Lithium was introduced into medicine in 1850 for the treatment of gout. During the following century many medical uses of lithium were proposed: as a stimulant, as a sedative, for the treatment of diabetes, for the treatment of infectious diseases, as an additive to tooth paste, for the treatment of malignant growths, etc. The efficacy of lithium in these conditions was not proved, and lithium treatment never became widespread. Use of lithium as a taste substitute in the low-salt diet of patients suffering from kidney and heart disease led to serious poisonings and induced fear of lithium in many physicians.

Discovery of the Therapeutic Effect in Mania

In 1949 an Australian psychiatrist, *John Cade,* published an article which forms the basis of all later lithium treatment. During the previous year he had carried out experiments with guinea pigs into which he injected urine and various chemicals to examine their toxicity. Among the chemicals were lithium salts, and he gained the impression that guinea pigs injected with these became quieter and responded less to stimuli but without becoming sleepy.

The idea then occurred to *Cade* that lithium might be better than the sedatives then in use for the treatment of violent psychiatric patients. He gave lithium salts to various patients, and in most there was no effect or very uncertain effect. However, in a small group of manic patients the symptoms disappeared within a week; they reappeared when treatment with lithium was discontinued.

Cade reported his observations in an Australian journal, but reactions were modest. In the years 1952–1954, this therapy was reinvestigated in the Psychiatric Clinic of Aarhus University in Risskov, Denmark. A so-called double-blind trial was carried out with a group of about 40 patients. They were given either active tablets or dummy tablets, that is tablets without lithium but otherwise similar to the lithium-containing tablets. This procedure was followed in order to distinguish between imagined effects and true treatment effects. The trial confirmed *John Cade's* observations; lithium was clearly active against manic agitation.

Discovery of the Prophylactic Effect in Recurrent
Manic-Depressive Illness

Attempts to treat depressive episodes of manic-depressive illness with lithium had given ambiguous results, and it was therefore unexpected when in 1959–1960 an English psychiatrist, *G.P. Hartigan,* and a Danish psychiatrist, *P.C. Baastrup,* observed that manic-depressive patients had fewer depressions or stopped having depressions when they were given long-term lithium treatment to keep manic attacks from occurring. *Poul Christian Baastrup* started a systematic treatment trial in the Psychiatric Hospital in Glostrup, Denmark. It was completed 6 years later in collaboration with the author of this book and involved long-term administration of lithium to patients with frequent relapses. The trial confirmed that this treatment in many cases led to fewer relapses of both mania and depression or to their complete disappearance. The effect is illustrated in figure 1, which is from a later follow-up study.

The prophylactic action of lithium in manic-depressive illness was debated in the psychiatric literature for some years, but extensive trials in many countries have now fully documented the efficacy of the drug. Its prophylactic action is exerted against both manic and depressive relapses, and it can be seen in unipolar patients as well as in bipolar patients. Lithium is now being used extensively. Sales figures for lithium preparations and reports from lithium clinics indicate that, in countries such as Denmark, Norway, Sweden, England, Canada and the United States, 1–1.5 persons out of every 1,000 in the population are under lithium treatment.

Lithium Treatment of Mania

It is characteristic of lithium treatment that it removes the manic symptoms without producing sedation. This is different from treatment with neuroleptics, which are also active in mania, but which exert sedative action. An experienced patient, who under previous manic episodes had tried both neuroleptics and lithium, reported that during treatment with the former he felt as if the brake and the gas pedal were pressed down at the same time. Lithium treatment gave the impression that the ignition key had been turned off.

Lithium may occasionally produce side effects: nausea, stomach ache, tremor of the hands, muscle weakness, etc., but usually they do not trouble the manic patients. The greatest drawback of the treatment is that the full antimanic effect usually is not seen until after 6–8 days of treatment, and sometimes it is necessary to supplement with a neuroleptic drug.

Fig. 1. Showing the disease course of manic-depressive patients treated with lithium. Each horizontal line of symbols corresponds to a patient's disease course from 1st January 1960 to 1st July 1969. The black rectangles are depressions, the vertically striped ones manias, and those with oblique lines are mixed states. The slim horizontal line indicates lithium treatment. The figure shows how prolonged lithium treatment led to a fall in the frequency of relapses. Many patients did not have further attacks after lithium treatment had been started. Some patients had relapses during lithium treatment but in most cases less frequently than before treatment. Some patients suffered relapse when, against the doctor's advice, they stopped lithium. From *Schou:* Die Lithiumprophylaxe bei manisch-depressiven Psychosen. *Nervenarzt,* vol. 42, pp. 1–10, 1971.

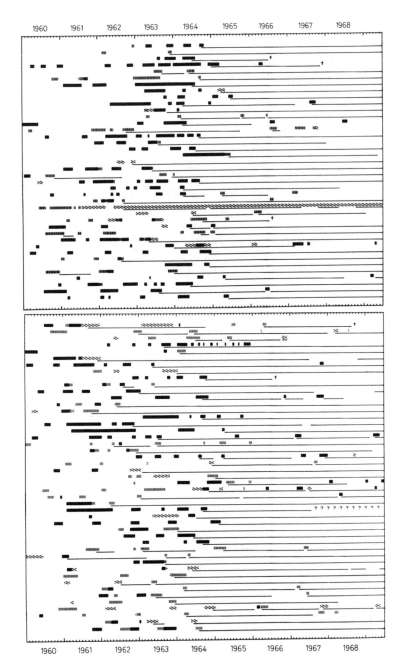

In mild or moderately severe mania, lithium is better than any other treatment. As the symptoms are not severe, the slow onset of the effect does not create great problems, and the 'soft' lithium effect is more pleasant for the patients than the effect of other medicine.

If a mania has become severe and the patient exhibits violence, restlessness, temper outbursts, etc., lithium may initially be combined with a quickacting sedative. Within the first week the dosage of the sedative is reduced gradually, and hereafter treatment is continued with lithium alone.

If the patient has had many previous attacks of mania and depression, there may be an indication for prophylactic treatment. In this instance lithium intake continues so that therapy leads directly into prophylaxis. If, on the other hand, the patient experiences his first episode or has had only few earlier episodes, lithium may be discontinued after 2–4 months.

Lithium Treatment against the Patient's Wish?

Due to lack of insight the manic patient may object to lithium treatment. It is, however, not possible to force patients to swallow lithium tablets, and in my opinion it is not advisable to administer lithium secretly by mixing crushed tablets with the food. Under these circumstances there is insufficient control of dosage and serum lithium concentration, and drug treatment of a person without his or her acceptance may compromise confidence between patient and relatives. It may also present ethical and legal problems.

Treatments other than lithium may have to be given, for instance a neuroleptic applied as an injection, until the patient improves and can accept lithium administration.

Lithium Treatment of Depression

Lithium may be used for the treatment of manic episodes and for the prevention of manic and depressive episodes; the prophylactic effect is almost equally good against depressions and against manias.

Lithium may also be used for treatment of the depressive episode itself, but this use is less widespread, because treatment with antidepressants and electric convulsive treatment all in all seem to be more effective. Depressions that have not yielded to treatment with antidepressant drugs may respond when lithium is added, the so-called augmentation treatment.

Prophylactic Lithium Treatment

Prophylaxis means prevention, but lithium cannot prevent the development of manic-depressive illness. Lithium prophylaxis is to be understood as prevention of relapse, so that manic and depressive recurrences become fewer or disappear during the treatment. Prophylactic lithium treatment keeps the illness under control, but it does not cure it. If the patient stops taking lithium, the disease is likely to reappear with episodes as frequent and severe as before. It is therefore necessary that patients continue taking lithium also during periods when no signs of illness are present.

For Whom Is Prophylactic Lithium Treatment Indicated?

Prophylactic lithium treatment should generally be given only to patients with manic-depressive illness and with repeated episodes. Opinions differ as to how frequent episodes should be to constitute grounds for start of long-term treatment with lithium. Patients who have had 2–3 episodes within the last 2–3 years are often given lithium prophylactically, but the treatment may also be considered when a patient has a new episode within 3–4 years after the occurrence of the previous episode. Studies from recent years have shown that under these circumstances there is risk of further relapses.

However, such rules serve only as crude guidelines. The individual patient's disease course, disease intensity, and life situation must be taken into account. Frequent episodes within recent years, severe depressions with suicide attempts, violent manias with destructive effects on marriage and economy, poor effect of traditional treatment, all these factors indicate that lithium treatment may be of use. Family and social conditions play a role; prophylactic treatment may, for example, be given before and during an important examination when a manic or depressive relapse would be particularly deleterious. It is important that the patients are co-responsible for deciding about prophylactic lithium treatment, and they should be given full and sober information about its advantages and disadvantages.

Lithium prophylaxis is not always effective. Out of ten patients treated, one or two may not respond, three or four may respond only partially, and four or five may respond fully.

Start of Treatment

Prophylactic lithium treatment may be started during a mania, during a depression, or during an interval. The last is presumably the most frequent. Lithium may be taken concurrently with antidepressant medication.

In some patients the prophylactic effect of lithium sets in immediately; they simply do not experience any further relapses. In other patients the prophylactic effect develops gradually, for example over a half to 1 year, and this slow onset is something of a riddle. The explanation can hardly be that the lithium concentration in the brain must equilibrate with that in the blood, because this is achieved within less than a week. Other biological explanations have been considered, for example slow readjustment of metabolic processes, but the explanation may also be psychological. When patients are unaccustomed to being in prophylactic treatment, they may forget to take the tablets, and they may have to experience relapses before they learn to take the medicine regularly.

Patients who do not suffer actual episodes during treatment occasionally experience what may be called 'reminders', single days or a week when they feel as if a depressive attack was underway without this actually developing.

Supplementary Drug Treatment

If mania develops during prophylactic lithium treatment, the lithium dosage is increased temporarily or lithium is supplemented with a sedative drug. Occurrence of depressive relapse may necessitate treatment with antidepressant drugs or electric convulsive treatment together with lithium if the depression is severe. However, the depressions that occur during lithium treatment are often mild and last only a few weeks, and it is gratifying for both patient and physician if they manage to weather the storm without taking recourse to extra medical treatment.

Alternative Prophylactic Treatments

If lithium proves to be ineffective in patients with frequent and severe episodes, alternative prophylactic drug treatment may be considered.

As mentioned above, prolonged administration of antidepressant drugs exerts a certain protection against new depressive episodes, and in patients with a unipolar course the choice between prophylactic treatment with antidepressants and prophylactic treatment with lithium may depend on how the patients tolerate the two treatments. Patients with a bipolar course are apt to develop new manic episodes when given long-term treatment with antidepressants.

For bipolar patients the antiepileptic drugs valproate and, in particular, carbamazepine seem to be valid alternatives, either given alone or in combination with lithium.

Does Lithium Gradually Lose Its Effect?

A number of drugs lose their effect when they have been used for some time; bigger doses must be given or treatment must be interrupted for some time in order to regain the previous effect. Lithium does not resemble these drugs. Even when it has been given for years, it seems to retain its full effect.

How Long Should Lithium Treatment Continue?

Lithium treatment is started in patients who have had several relapses over the last years, and treatment should often be given for years. This does not mean that patients are bound to lithium once they have started the treatment. It can be discontinued at any time if it does not prove effective or if side effects become troublesome.

There are patients who must continue with lithium for many years to remain free of relapses, but there are also those who need lithium only for a limited number of years. Patients with a unipolar course seem to have a better chance of stopping lithium with impunity after some years than patients with both manias and depressions. If a patient has been entirely free of relapses for 3–4 years, patient and physician may consider discontinuation of treatment under close supervision. In case of relapse, treatment is started again.

Abrupt discontinuation of lithium has in some patients led to transitory tenseness and restlessness. It is not clear whether these are abstinence phenomena or whether they are caused by removal of a weak sedative lithium action. It may be advisable to stop lithium by lowering the dosage gradually.

Lithium Pauses

The question has been raised whether patients on prophylactic lithium treatment may take a pause occasionally, for example for some months. This involves some risk, especially if the patients previously had frequent episodes.

The situation may be different for the small group of manic-depressive patients who have season-bound manias and depressions, for example relapses every winter or spring. In such cases it may seem tempting to stop lithium early in the summer and start again in late fall. But there are problems with this strategy. First, the seasonal rhythm of the disease may have changed during the treatment. Secondly, in some patients it takes some time before the full prophylactic effect develops, and prophylaxis may therefore be insufficient if the treatment is started too late. The technique of lithium pauses has not been explored enough, and I tend to advise against it.

Peeping under the Cover

To be freed of depressions is a clear advantage. To have manias removed can be a mixed blessing; some patients miss the manic episodes. It is therefore worth discussing a question which has been raised by patients who, in spite of good prophylactic lithium effect, occasionally feel a mania in progress under the cover of the treatment. Is it possible for such patients to lower the lithium dosage just so much that the mania develops to a pleasant extent but yet remains under control? I know that a few patients have done so and have utilized the excess energy and indefatigability of the mania to finish a particular piece of work, but I must warn against the procedure. Manias are like volcanos rather than boiling kettles, and once the forces are let loose, they may overpower the patient who perhaps loses insight and hence control over the tablet intake.

When Should Lithium Not Be Given?

Lithium treatment acts on manic-depressive illness, and lithium should generally not be given to patients who do not suffer from this disease. There are many other forms of depression than that which is part of manic-depressive illness, for example psychogenic depression or depressive lowering of mood as part of a neurosis; lithium is not effective in these conditions. A specialist in psychiatry must decide whether the patient suffers from manic-depressive illness; it is incorrect to start prophylactic lithium treatment merely because there have been depressive symptoms.

Lithium should not be given to patients with severe kidney disease, serious heart disease, or diseases with disturbance of fluid or salt balance. Liver disease as, for example, previous hepatitis with or without jaundice is without significance. One should be cautious about starting lithium treatment in patients with mild kidney disease, with elevated blood pressure, or with gastrointestinal infection, as well as in patients on a low-salt diet, in treatment with diuretics, or on a slimming diet. If a decision to start lithium treatment is nevertheless made, the therapy should be carried out under careful control.

Kidney function falls with advancing age, but this does not mean that old people may not have lithium. They should merely be given lower doses, and usually the lithium concentration in the blood should be kept somewhat lower than in younger persons.

Lithium Treatment of Conditions Other than Manic-Depressive Illness

Lithium treatment has been tried in diseases other than manic-depressive illness. The trials are outside the scope of this book, but it may be mentioned that lithium occasionally is of value in patients who suffer from both schizophrenia and manic-depressive illness. In such cases lithium treatment may provide stabilization, especially when combined with a neuroleptic drug. Lithium has also been tried in cases of long-lasting emotional instability in children and adolescents, for sudden impulsive aggressiveness in persons of unstable character, for severe depressive symptoms before menstruation, for alcoholism, and in a number of physical diseases. In most of the conditions lithium treatment has been without effect or without clear-cut effect.

It should perhaps be emphasized that lithium exerts its action against abnormal mania and depression. It is no good taking lithium because one has become angry or in the hope of relieving grief.

How Does Lithium Work?

Lithium has a very large number of biological effects, and this has presumably to do with the fact that it resembles the naturally occurring ions sodium, potassium, calcium, and magnesium. Lithium exerts actions on the cell wall, on

23

impulse transmission, on hormone reactions, on metabolic processes, and much more. It is, however, difficult to decide which effect or effects are related to the action of lithium in manic-depressive illness, because the causes of this disease are still unknown. It is unlikely that manic-depressive illness is caused by lithium deficiency. Lithium may regulate a brain mechanism which is out of balance during mania or depression and which is easily brought out of balance in persons with a predisposition for manic-depressive illness. It is possible that lithium increases mental resistance to those, still unknown, external and internal influences which precipitate attacks of mania and depression. Perhaps lithium brings a disturbed rhythm function in the organism under control. These and many other hypotheses are under examination, and new knowledge is acquired continuously.

5 On Being in Lithium Treatment

Gains

In the section 'On Being Manic-Depressive' I described how manic-depressive illness may interfere with the life and well-being of patient and family, how disease attacks may lead to destruction and grief, and how intervals may become dominated by uncertainty, tension, and fear of the future.

All this is altered by successful lithium prophylaxis. Relapses become few and mild and may disappear completely. The patients once more become the persons they were before the disease started. Spouses describe how the patient is now 'on an even keel', 'in much better shape than he has been for years', 'able to cope with difficult situations much more adequately', 'again her own self as she was when we married', etc.

After years in the shadow of fear it may be difficult to hope again, but gradually patient and family experience how the disease course has been changed and how the fear loses its grip. The patient feels that life once more becomes safe and predictable and that normal relationships can be established or re-established. A patient wrote, 'Above all it is gratifying to be trusted, and that people around you start making normal demands'. For patients whose existence was dominated by frequent and severe manic-depressive relapses, treatment with lithium may improve life quality miraculously.

Problems

Lithium treatment is accordingly of undoubted value for many persons. Why is it then that sometimes it arouses mixed or angry feelings in patients and relatives? Why do patients occasionally neglect tablet intake? And why do some patients stop treatment entirely? These questions cannot be answered simply and clearly, but there is reason to examine them, so that the patients and their doctors can take them up for discussion.

There may be many reasons why patients are dissatisfied with lithium treatment and perhaps want to stop it. The most obvious is presumably that it does not work or does not work as well as the patient had expected and hoped. Perhaps treatment was started on the basis of a wrong diagnosis. Perhaps the patient had expected a one hundred percent efficacy or hoped that the treatment would solve all personal and marital problems. Perhaps there are factors in the patient's life which maintain the disease pattern and the patient role. Perhaps the patient does not want to miss the well-being and increased self-confidence of the mild manias. Perhaps the patient does not take the tablets regularly. Perhaps the treatment has not been given for a sufficiently long time. Patient and physician must discuss the problems and decide whether treatment should be stopped or whether it should be continued, possibly with altered dosage.

There are also instances where patients stop taking lithium because they feel well. There have been no relapses for a long time, and they think that lithium treatment is no longer necessary. This may or may not be the case; at any rate patient and doctor should discuss the matter.

There are patients who have difficulty accepting that they must be in long-term treatment. They dislike the idea that their mental health and emotional balance are regulated by a drug on which, in a way, they therefore become dependent. This is admittedly not drug dependence in the traditional sense of the word, development of craving and habit formation, but the very necessity of having to take medicine every day may give a feeling of being bound.

'An effort is required to live with the lithium treatment', wrote a patient. She was thinking of the obligatory daily tablet intake but also of problems posed by the curiosity and uncertainty of people noticing the consumption of medicine. Some patients choose to be open about their manic-depressive illness and lithium treatment ('Those who reject you may not be worth knowing!'), but others prefer, perhaps taught by bitter experiences, to keep the disease a secret and to take the tablets when nobody watches. The same correspondent described how family attitudes sometimes maintain the patient in a disease pattern even after lithium has brought the disease under control. 'Mental toughness is required to go against the expectations of your family.'

Some patients feel that lithium treatment changes their personality and reactions. Life is greyer than before, there is less enthusiasm, energy, and resolution, mental and physical reactions are not as quick as they used to be, nor memory as astute. Part of the mechanism underlying these experiences may be that lithium has prevented or weakened manic elation, and there are patients who express very clearly that they miss the surplus and productivity of the mild manias. It is, however, also possible that in some patients lithium may affect or inhibit normal mental functions and produce a feeling of personality change. There are patients who experience relief after discontinuation of lithium or reduction of dosage, because they feel that their ordinary self returns.

It is not always the elation that is missed. An undertaker was blamed for his apparent lack of compassion after lithium had removed his slight depressions. Another patient regretted that in discussions he was no longer able to obtain the level of excitement which he considered necessary, commenting, 'Doctor, I am a politician, and I *must* get excited when I discuss'.

Patients may also want to stop the treatment because they have side effects, especially if these are severe and the prophylactic effect of the treatment not very good. Patient and physician must weigh gains and losses. Particularly troublesome side effects may be weight gain, hand tremor with affection of the handwriting, thirst and frequent urination, occasionally eruption of psoriasis.

For the patient's family and friends a feeling of immense relief is in almost all cases the dominant reaction to the result of successful lithium treatment. But those who are close to the patient may need time to adjust to the new situation. This is best illustrated by the effect of lithium on marital relations. In most cases the marital climate is markedly improved during lithium treatment, but occasionally the spouse misses the enthusiasm and sexual intensity which the patient previously showed during mild manias.

Successful lithium prophylaxis also leads to a radical reshuffling of roles and responsibilities in the family. The main sufferer under this is the spouse, whose central role as upholder of home and family is endangered by the patient's recovery and who therefore may sabotage the treatment secretly or openly. Patient, spouse, and doctor must work together with these problems.

Lithium and Creative Work

Patients occasionally assert that lithium treatment lowers their flow of ideas, fantasy, and productivity, and that their creative ability has become weakened. These are serious disadvantages for persons whose professional work is based on the ability to generate ideas and to translate them into practical or scientific or artistic productivity. However, long-term lithium treatment is given to persons with frequent episodes of mania or depression or both, and these attacks may in themselves affect creative work. The question is therefore: What is worse, the disease or the treatment?

In order to obtain an impression of advantages and disadvantages I contacted a number of manic-depressive artists whose disease had been brought under control by lithium and asked them: What happened to your creative ability? Out of 24 artists six reported that their productivity had remained unaltered. Six others felt that ideas now came less readily and that their productivity had declined during lithium treatment; four of them stopped lithium for this reason. They preferred to maintain the inspiration and energy of the mild manias and were in return willing to risk depressions and severe manias. There were finally 12 artists who felt that they created more and in some cases better during lithium treatment than before. Their depressions had been painful and artistically barren, their manias dominated by valueless overactivity. When lithium brought the disease under control, they could function with steadiness and better artistic discipline to the advantage of both the quantity and the quality of their work.

Collaboration between Patient and Physician
The Patient's Own Responsibility

Prophylactic lithium treatment places a responsibility on both patient and physician, and they must collaborate in order to achieve best possible treatment results. Persons in prophylactic treatment are not 'ill', and they should try to replace the passive patient role with active effort for their own benefit. Lithium treatment has a better chance of giving good results if the patients study treatment guidelines and follow them closely. It requires resolution to adjust to the new life under lithium and to re-establish relationships with family and friends, and extra courage and endurance are needed if the illness occasionally shows signs of returning. Support from the family is of major importance.

Prophylactic lithium treatment makes demands on the physician's knowledge and care. Occasionally patients with many years of experience know more about manic-depressive illness and lithium than the physician who monitors the treatment, but it shows responsibility and is no shame if the physician asks for time to read more about the subject. This book is addressed also to physicians, and at the end of the book is a list of supplementary reading.

In most cases lithium treatment does not present any major medical or psychological problems, and contact between patient and physician may then be limited to relatively short consultations in connection with the laboratory controls. But the doctor's interest must include the patient's welfare and subjective experiences during the treatment, positive as well as negative, and if problems arise, they must be taken up for discussion. Sometimes it is advantageous to combine lithium treatment with regular psychotherapy. Group therapy and family therapy may also be considered.

It is important for the patient to know that the doctor is available and has time if problems arise. The contact person may also be a nurse, a psychologist, or a social worker who has experience with manic-depressive illness and with lithium treatment. Special help may be provided by other patients who are or have been in lithium treatment. Exchange of experiences in the waiting room of a lithium clinic may be of considerable value, and patients in lithium treatment can meet in clubs in order to discuss problems and share experiences.

6 Practical Management of the Treatment

Preparations

Lithium may be taken as tablets, as capsules, or in the form of a syrup. Table 1 shows preparations marketed in English-speaking countries.

Two of the preparations contain lithium citrate, the others lithium carbonate, but this does not matter much because it is the lithium ion which is active. It is more important that different preparations have different lithium contents; change from one preparation to another may therefore require change in number of tablets in order to retain the lithium dosage, expressed in millimoles per day, at the same level. Some of the preparations are so-called slow-release or controlled-release tablets; they release lithium more gradually in the intestine and should be swallowed, not crushed or chewed.

It does not matter much whether lithium is taken with a meal, but the tablets should be washed down with ample amounts of fluid. Occasionally patients have difficulty in swallowing tablets or capsules, and a lithium-containing syrup may be preferred. Another possibility is to take the tablets in yoghurt. It is not essential that the tablets are taken at exactly the same time each day, but on the day preceding blood control the last dose should be taken 12 hours (between 11 and 13 hours) before the blood sample is drawn.

Lithium preparations are best stored in a dry place and out of direct sunlight. They must be kept out of reach of children.

Some patients find it difficult to remember to take their tablets, at least until they have established a treatment routine. We are dealing with a prophylactic treatment, and there are accordingly no symptoms to remind the patients of the tablets. It may be an advantage to use clear plastic containers with separate compartments for each day of the week. If the container is filled on a particular weekday, there is not much to remember during the week, and it is possible to see at a glance whether any tablet intake has been forgotten. If a tablet has been forgotten, the patient should not try to make up by taking more tablets the next time. One or two omissions usually do not matter.

Table 1. Lithium preparations marketed in English-speaking countries

Name	Drug company	Lithium salt	Amount of salt mg	Amount of lithium mmol	Type
Camcolit-400	Norgine, England	carbonate	400	10.8	slow-release
Carbolith	ICN, Canada	carbonate	300	8.1	conventional
Cibalith-S	Ciba, USA	citrate	752 in 5 ml	8.0 in 5 ml	syrup
Eskalith	Smith Kline & French, USA	carbonate	300	8.1	conventional
Eskalith CR	Smith Kline & French, USA	carbonate	300	8.1	slow-release
Liskonum	Smith Kline & French, England	carbonate	450	12.2	slow-release
Litarex	CD, England	citrate	564	6.0	slow-release
Lithane	Pfizer, Canada	carbonate	300	8.1	conventional
Lithicarb	Protea, Australia	carbonate	250	6.8	conventional
Lithium Carbonate	Roxane, USA	carbonate	150/300/600	4.0/8.1/16.2	conventional
Lithium Phasal	Pharmax, England	carbonate	300	8.1	slow-release
Lithizine	Paul Maney, Canada	carbonate	150/300	4.0/8.1	conventional
Lithobid	Ciba, USA	carbonate	300	8.1	slow-release
Lithonate	Reid-Rowell, USA	carbonate	300	8.1	conventional
Lithotabs	Reid-Rowell, USA	carbonate	300	8.1	conventional
Manialith	Muir & Neil, Australia	carbonate	250	6.8	conventional
Priadel	Delandale, England, and Protea, Australia	carbonate	400	10.8	slow-release
Priadel Liquid	Delandale, England	citrate	520 in 5 ml	5.5 in 5 ml	syrup

The author has tried to provide exact information, but he cannot be held responsible for any errors in or omissions from the table.

Laboratory Examinations

Before lithium treatment is started, the patient is examined by the physician and interviewed about previous or present illnesses. Laboratory examinations are carried out to check the physical condition. Such tests may include examination of the urine and determination of serum creatinine, sedimentation rate, and thyroid-stimulating hormone in serum (serum TSH). Also advisable are measurement of blood pressure, an electrocardiogram, and measurement of body weight. Depending on the patient's age, condition, previous illness, etc., further examinations may be needed.

During treatment with lithium the patient is followed with regular laboratory examinations. The most important tests are determinations of serum lithium, serum creatinine, and serum-TSH, but further tests may be required.

The serum lithium concentration is determined once a week during the first weeks in order to assist dosage adjustment. Thereafter determinations are carried out every 2–4 months or at longer intervals as agreed between patient and physician. Attention is directed particularly towards unexpected changes of the concentration. A consistent rise of serum lithium with unchanged dosage or a disproportionate rise after dosage increase may indicate that lithium is excreted less effectively by the kidneys, and it may be necessary to subject the patient's drug intake, dietary habits, and kidney function to closer examination. The lithium concentration is determined in blood samples drawn 12 hours (11–13 hours) after the last lithium dose. If a longer or shorter time has elapsed, the patient should report this. The blood samples are usually drawn from a vein in the elbow, but some laboratories are equipped with such sensitive flame photometers that they only require blood from a prick in the ear or the finger. The patients need not be fasting.

The serum creatinine concentration is determined in order to monitor kidney function. Lithium is excreted almost exclusively through the kidneys, and it is therefore important that any kidney disease with lowered kidney function is detected early. Attention is drawn to changes in the serum creatinine concentration rather than to absolute values because a consistent rise of serum creatinine may indicate lowered kidney function, even if the concentration is below the upper limit of the normal range. Serum creatinine is determined together with serum lithium.

Serum TSH may be determined every 6–12 months in order to assist in the detection of early changes of thyroid function.

Patients in lithium treatment may serve as blood donors.

The frequency of control visits is usually determined by clinical considerations. It is important for the cooperation between patient and doctor that they meet at intervals to discuss treatment progress, and the main importance of the laboratory visits may lie in the provision of a structured framework for these contacts. Intervals between routine checkups therefore depend on the patient's personality and conscientiousness, the extent of information and instruction given, the clinic routine, etc.

Recommendations given here deal with minimum requirements for laboratory monitoring under ordinary circumstances. But sometimes such 'ordinary' circumstances are extraordinary. In developing countries even strongly indicated lithium treatment may not be instituted because laboratory facilities are lacking, and in countries without a socialized health system poor patients may be deprived of this treatment because they cannot afford the cost of regular laboratory examinations. In my opinion it is not irresponsible for a doctor to prescribe lithium treatment even without laboratory monitoring, if the alternative is that no prophylactic therapy is given.

Dosage Adjustment in Prophylactic Lithium Treatment

During prophylactic lithium treatment a dosage should be used which gives protection against manic and depressive relapses and has as few side effects as possible. In some cases side effects cannot be entirely avoided. The dosage requirement differs for different patients, and the daily lithium dosage may vary from about 6–8 mmol to about 70–80 mmol. Frequently used prophylactic doses are 20–30 mmol daily.

There are two reasons why dosage requirements differ. First, different patients excrete lithium with different rates so that they require different doses to achieve the same serum lithium concentration. Second, the sensitivity of different patients to lithium may differ, so that different patients must be adjusted to slightly different serum lithium levels. Since the patients' sensitivity and excretion rate are not known in advance, dosage adjustment is a stepwise process, and table 2 shows a proposed procedure which falls in three steps or phases.

Phase 1: During the first week a lithium dosage is administered which is so low that it will be harmless even to patients with high sensitivity and low excretion rate. A daily dosage of 6–8 mmol is appropriate.

Phase 2: After 1 week the serum lithium concentration is determined, and the dosage is adjusted to a standard serum lithium level of 0.5–0.8 mmol/l. This

33

Table 2. Proposed procedure for dosage adjustment during prophylactic lithium treatment

---

Phase 1

Treatment is started with a low dose, for example 1 tablet daily

---

Phase 2

After one week the serum lithium concentration is determined and the dosage adjusted (dosage and serum lithium are directly proportional) to a serum lithium level of 0.5–0.8 mmol/l. Serum lithium is determined at weekly intervals during the following 2 weeks, and if necessary the dosage is readjusted

---

Phase 3

If with serum lithium at 0.5–0.8 mmol/l manic or depressive relapses still occur, the dosage is raised slightly and the patient maintained at the new and higher serum lithium level.

If with serum lithium at 0.5–0.8 mmol/l side effects are troublesome, the dosage is reduced slightly and the patient maintained at the new and lower serum lithium level

---

Throughout the treatment

Attention is at all times paid to *changes* of serum lithium. A consistent rise of serum lithium with unaltered dosage or a disproportionate rise after a dosage increase signals a fall of renal lithium clearance and requires further examination

---

level usually provides good prophylactic effect and relatively few side effects. There is direct proportionality between dosage and serum lithium so that a doubling of dosage leads to a doubling of serum lithium. Determinations of serum lithium during the following weeks serve to check that the required level has been reached.

Phase 3: In some patients the occurrence of relapses or the development of troublesome side effects may necessitate adjustment of the dosage to serum lithium levels outside the standard range. There are patients who do not tolerate and do not need serum lithium concentrations higher than 0.3–0.4 mmol/l, while other patients can be protected effectively against manic and depressive relapses only if their serum lithium is between 0.8 and 1.0 mmol/l. Serum lithium concentrations lower than 0.3 mmol/l are inactive in most patients, and serum concentrations over 1.0 mmol/l are often accompanied by serious side effects and may involve risk of poisoning.

It must be remembered that insufficient response to lithium treatment may have other causes than too low dosages and serum lithium concentrations: negligent tablet intake, insufficient treatment duration, psychological complications, etc. The patient's total situation must be taken into consideration when measures against insufficient treatment effect are considered.

Type of Preparation and Number of Daily Doses

Slow-release preparations release lithium more gradually in the intestines than do conventional tablets, and this results in narrower variations of the serum lithium concentration. Serum lithium also varies less widely when lithium is given in two or three daily doses than when it is given in a single dose in the evening.

It has been debated whether it is best to take one or two daily doses and whether conventional or slow-release tablets are best. These seem, however, to be factors of minor significance. The most important procedure for avoiding or counteracting side effects is to use as low doses and serum concentrations as are compatible with satisfactory treatment response. If particular side effects remain troublesome, one may try to change the lithium preparation or the number of daily doses.

It is rarely necessary to use more than two daily doses, but if distribution of the daily dosage on three intakes is tolerated best, it is preferable that the tablets are taken in the morning, late in the afternoon, and at bedtime. Experience shows that tablet intake during working hours is easily forgotten.

7 Side Effects

Lithium treatment is often accompanied by side effects. They are in many cases not troublesome, and they may appear for a brief period only. But the side effects may also become so troublesome and unpleasant that the patients choose to stop treatment because they find that these unwanted side effects outweigh any advantages.

Sometimes lithium is blamed without justification. When a treatment is given on a long-term basis, it almost automatically becomes the scape-goat when things go wrong. Patients are inclined to blame the medication for any ailment or unpleasantness they may experience, be it headache or sleeplessness or stomach ulcer, and the same happens when the patients do not feel in optimum form, not so happy and energetic as they would like to be or as they feel they are entitled to be. Lithium shares this fate with other long-term medications.

Side Effects at the Start of Treatment

Start of lithium treatment is often associated with side effects during the first 1–2 weeks: nausea, stomach ache, loose stools, and a feeling of fatigue in arms and legs. The organism eventually gets used to the drug, and these side effects usually disappear on continued treatment.

Hand Tremor

In some patients lithium produces tremor of the hands within the first 1–2 years of the treatment; thereafter it usually disappears. It is an aggravation of the light tremor which most people experience at times and which may be more pronounced in some families. In most cases the tremor is so weak that it is scarcely perceived, but some patients may find it troublesome if their vocation requires a steady hand (surgeon, watchmaker), or they may be embarrassed at parties when the coffee cup rattles in the saucer or when they must grip the glass with both hands in order not to spill the contents. Patients who take lithium and antidepressant drugs concurrently are particularly tremor-prone.

The tremor may change during the day and become worse when the patient is tired or tense, or after smoking or consumption of caffeine-containing beverages (coffee, tea, cola). The development of marked and irregular tremor can be a sign of impending intoxication.

Troublesome tremor may be counteracted by reducing the lithium dosage and the serum lithium level. It may also be useful to change from conventional lithium tablets to the slow-release type and from one daily dose to two or three. If these procedures are insufficient, it may be possible to reduce the tremor by concurrent intake of a 'beta-blocking agent' such as propranolol (Inderal) or pindolol (Viskén). It is often sufficient to take 10–20 mg of the drug half an hour before the meeting or party where tremor would be inconvenient.

A few patients are bothered by reduced reaction speed and precision in quick ball games such as table tennis or squash. In other patients the handwriting may become less legible.

Effect on the Heart

Changes of the function or electrical activity of the heart are occasionally seen during lithium treatment, but the presence of heart disease rarely prevents well-motivated lithium treatment of manic-depressive illness. In case of heart disease the question of lithium treatment should be discussed with a cardiologist, and the treatment may have to be monitored with special care, for example with repeated electrocardiograms.

Effect on the Thyroid Gland

During lithium treatment the thyroid gland may increase in size with swelling of the neck (goiter), or thyroid function may decrease with the result that metabolism is lowered (myxedema). The neck swelling is usually discovered by the family or because the patient feels that his shirt collar is too tight. Myxedema is more easily missed, because some of its symptoms resemble a slight depression: tiredness, lowered vitality, sadness, slow reactions, in some cases thickening of the skin and a feeling of coldness. Determinations of the thyroid-stimulating hormone (TSH) in blood serum can be a support for the diagnosis, because this laboratory value rises to abnormal levels at an early stage, possibly before there are clear signs in the patient's condition.

Once lithium-induced goiter or myxedema have been discovered, they are easy to treat. Thyroid hormone (thyroxine) or related preparations are taken together with lithium. The gland then shrinks to its normal size, and the signs of myxedema disappear. The treatment is simple, safe and effective.

Effect on the Kidneys

Lithium is excreted almost exclusively through the kidneys, and their function is therefore of decisive importance for the treatment. Concern was generated some years ago when microscopy of kidney tissue samples indicated that structural changes could occur in the kidneys of lithium-treated patients. Did this mean that prolonged lithium treatment might eventually damage the kidneys and lead to kidney insufficiency? This fear has proved unfounded. Extensive examinations of large patient groups have shown that lithium treatment does not lead to gradual destruction of the kidneys and kidney insufficiency, not even when lithium is given for many years.

Lithium treatment may affect one particular function of the kidneys, water excretion, but that has been known for many years. The human kidney works in sections. In the first section large amounts of very dilute urine are produced, several hundred liters per day, but in later sections the urine is concentrated through absorption of water back into the blood stream, and normally only ½–2 liters of urine are excreted per day, the volume depending on individual drinking habits. During lithium treatment the ability to concentrate the urine may become impaired, so that more urine than normal is excreted, for example 2–4 liters daily, in some cases up to 6–8 liters or more.

The increased urine formation is called polyuria. Patients suffering from this side effect must urinate frequently; this may disturb sleep during the night and cause social embarrassment during the day. The increased loss of fluid necessitates increased fluid intake (polydipsia). The patients become thirsty quickly and must drink often. If they do not drink for some hours, they may become unwell. Consumption of large amounts of calorie-rich beverages may lead to weight gain as an extra side effect, and a large beer intake may lead to alcoholism.

Patients with lithium-induced polyuria are at particular risk of becoming dehydrated if they do not consume sufficient amounts of fluid.

The best way of counteracting the effect of lithium on water excretion is to use low dosages and maintain low serum lithium levels. Impaired concentrating ability occurs much less frequently when serum lithium is maintained below 0.8 mmol/l than when it is higher. Pronounced polyuria may be treated with diuretic drugs, but the treatment is not without risk and should be carried out under careful monitoring. After discontinuation of lithium treatment the kidneys regain their concentrating ability, but this may take some months.

Effect on the Skin

In rare cases lithium treatment may lead to skin changes, for example appearance or aggravation of acne (pimples) or psoriasis. They usually disappear when treatment is stopped.

Effect on the Stomach and the Intestine

During the days after start of lithium treatment, but in some cases also later, stomach ache and nausea may occur, and the intestinal function may be affected. The stools become looser, and there may be a sudden urge to defecate. In such cases it may be an advantage to change from slow-release tablets to conventional tablets or vice versa.

Edema

Transitory formation of edema (swelling due to accumulation of fluid in the tissues) is not infrequent in patients given lithium. It may be localized in the legs, the hands, the abdominal wall, and occasionally the face. Usually the edema disappears after a short time, but it may persist longer. In this situation it is tempting to start treatment with diuretics, but as emphasized already such treatment should be carried out under careful monitoring.

Weight Gain

Many manic-depressive patients have experienced weight gain during treatment with antidepressants or neuroleptics; the same phenomenon may be seen during lithium treatment. Alteration of the metabolism or of the appetite regulating center in the brain may play a role, but in the case of lithium there may also be weight gain due to quenching of lithium-induced thirst with calorie-rich beverages such as beer, milk and soft drinks.

The weight gain usually occurs within the first 6–12 months of the treatment; after this the body weight stabilizes. Patients who are already overweight and patients taking lithium and antidepressants together are more prone to gain weight and should pay particular attention to appropriate exercise and reduction of calorie intake.

Weight gain may be a troublesome side effect, and there are patients who interrupt treatment for this reason. The only effective counter-measure is a reduction of the intake of calories, and it is particularly important that thirst is quenched with water, tea without sugar, or sugar-free soft drinks. If patients try to lose weight through use of a slimming diet, they should take extra salt in order to avoid salt deficiency. Diet pills with stimulant properties should be avoided.

Effect on Mental Functions

The kind and frequency of mental side effects of lithium are subject to discussion, because manic-depressive illness itself may affect not only mood and activity but also the ability to think and remember, and it is sometimes difficult to distinguish between what is caused by lithium and what by the illness.

Psychological tests carried out in healthy volunteers before, during, and after lithium intake have in some cases revealed an effect on vigilance, memory, reaction time, etc., but for obvious reasons such experiments last only a short time, days or weeks, and the results cannot readily be applied to patients in long-lasting lithium treatment. More informative are psychological examinations carried out on patients in lithium treatment before and after temporary transference to dummy tablets. This led in some patients to manic or depressive relapse. Among the patients who did not relapse the tests occasionally showed improved memory for visual impressions and increased ability to perform complicated tasks based on visual impressions and reaction ability. There may be a connection between such test results and the feeling some lithium-treated patients have of impaired memory and lowered reaction speed and precision. In the section 'Problems' I described how some patients may feel that lithium treatment changes their personality. However, most patients feel normal and function normally during lithium treatment.

Lithium effects on mental functions are readily reversible and disappear when lithium is discontinued or the dosage reduced.

It should be remembered that slow reactions and impaired memory can be signs of depressive relapse or lowered thyroid gland function. If this is the case, appropriate treatment should be given.

Male patients occasionally complain of decreased sexual potency during lithium treatment, but it is not clear whether this is a lithium effect, a sign of slight depressive relapse, or a coincidence.

Car Driving?

It cannot be entirely excluded that lithium occasionally may affect reactions to such a degree that driving ability is impaired. It may be wise for patients starting lithium treatment to abstain from car driving until they have found out how much the treatment affects their coordination. I know of no instance where lithium treatment permanently prevented car driving.

Development of Dependence?

All drugs with effects on the brain are in principle under suspicion for inducing addiction and dependence, but more than 40 years of psychiatric experience have shown that lithium is a safe drug in this respect. However, even if lithium does not produce pharmacological dependence, some patients may after years of lithium treatment have developed a kind of psychological dependence on the treatment regimen, the treatment situation, and the therapist and may for this reason feel anxiety after discontinuation of lithium. This problem should be coped with by patient and physician together.

8 Risk Factors

Lithium is a potent drug. There is often a narrow margin between the effective treatment dose and one high enough to produce troublesome side effects and risk of poisoning. However, lithium is not capricious. Risk of poisoning arises in particular situations, and by avoiding these the patient may contribute to the safety of the treatment.

Poisoning

Lithium poisoning may be dangerous; severe poisoning has led to death or to brain damage with lasting disturbances of gait and speech. It is therefore important that lithium poisoning is detected as early as possible and treated quickly and effectively.

A patient with impending lithium poisoning becomes dull and sleepy, has difficulty concentrating, feels muscle weakness and heaviness of the limbs. The gait becomes unsteady, marked hand tremor and slight muscle twitches appear, particularly when the patient is about to fall asleep. Frequently the patient has difficulty speaking distinctly. There may be diarrhea and nausea with vomiting. Table 3 shows a list of the signs of impending lithium poisoning. If one or more of these signs become prominent, the doctor should be informed so that an examination can be arranged, including determination of the serum lithium concentration. If it is not possible to reach the doctor, lithium must be stopped temporarily.

A patient with fully developed poisoning is markedly apathetic, muscle twitches become more prominent, hand tremor irregular, and movements are uncoordinated. In severe poisoning the brain and the kidneys are primarily affected. The patients may be completely unconscious, but occasionally they respond to stimuli with grunts or head movements. They look ill, and epileptic seizures may occur. Sometimes the condition resembles cerebral hemorrhage. Urine production may stop.

Table 3. Signs of impending lithium poisoning

Dullness	Tremor of the lower jaw
Sleepiness	Muscle twitches
Difficulty concentrating	Indistinct speech
Muscle weakness	Nausea
Heaviness of the limbs	Stomach ache
Unsteady gait	Diarrhea
Marked hand tremor	

Appearance of one or more of these signs and symptoms *may* indicate that a lithium poisoning is under development. The physician should be contacted for closer examination.

A patient with impending lithium intoxication should stop the lithium intake and should drink abundantly in order to avoid dehydration. Unless the poisoning is very mild, a lithium-poisoned patient should be admitted to hospital, because the condition may deteriorate during the following days even after lithium has been stopped. Treatment consists in correction of fluid and salt imbalance and control of kidney function. Treatment with an artificial kidney machine may be required in order to remove lithium as quickly and as efficiently as possible.

Depressed patients have occasionally tried to commit suicide by swallowing many lithium tablets, usually without success. Poisoning caused by acute overdosage seems to be less dangerous, although hardly less unpleasant, than the gradually developing lithium intoxication.

Risk Situations

It is important for the excretion of lithium through the kidneys that the body is in balance as regards water and sodium (sodium ion, Na^+). Balance means equilibrium between intake and output. Negative balance is the result of too little intake in relation to output or too large output in relation to intake so that water deficiency (dehydration) or sodium deficiency (salt deficiency) develops.

Under normal circumstances the risk of dehydration and salt deficiency is not large, because the kidneys have a considerable capacity for retaining salt and water in the body. But patients in lithium treatment are in a special situation, because their kidneys may have a reduced ability to concentrate urine and to

Table 4. Risk situations during lithium treatment

Physical disease with fever	Low-salt diet
Vomiting and diarrhea	Slimming diet
Prolonged unconsciousness	Treatment with diuretics
Narcosis and surgery	Pregnancy and delivery

In these situations lithium treatment should be monitored with special care, and attention should be paid to signs of impending poisoning (table 3).

Table 5. Situations in which it may become necessary to administer fluid by infusion to patients in lithium treatment

When the patients vomit massively
When the patients are unconscious for many hours
When the patients are prevented from drinking because of surgery with narcosis the next day

retain sodium, and even moderate dehydrations and salt deficiencies, which in themselves would not be dangerous, may lead to less efficient excretion of lithium; if the lithium dosage is not reduced or the treatment stopped, lithium poisoning may develop.

Water Deficiency (Dehydration)

Table 4 shows situations which may lead to risk of dehydration or salt deficiency. Both water and salt are lost during heavy sweating, for example during physical illness with fever. Physically ill persons also drink and eat less. Vomiting and diarrhea may contribute to the development of dehydration and salt deficiency. In these situations the lithium treatment should be monitored with particular caution, extra salt and water should be given, and the lithium administration may have to be interrupted temporarily.

Patients in lithium treatment should be particularly attentive to situations with risk of dehydration and should drink ample amounts of fluid. They must not neglect feelings of thirst for any prolonged time, and they should be advised to carry extra fluid in situations when it is difficult to have something to drink, for example on long car trips.

Occasionally it may be necessary to give extra fluid by infusion, slow injection under the skin or in a vein (table 5). Such treatment may be necessary in lithium treated patients who are unconscious or who vomit massively or who are prevented from drinking because they have to undergo surgery under narcosis the next day. These situations may lead to dehydration if the patients are not given fluid by infusion. Not all anesthesiologists and surgeons may be aware of this, so it may be wise for patients in lithium treatment to draw attention to their special situation.

Salt Deficiency

Sodium is usually consumed as sodium chloride, ordinary table salt, and the importance of the salt balance for lithium's excretion was illustrated dramatically in 1949 when, as mentioned previously, patients with kidney and heart disease given a low-salt diet were permitted to 'salt' their food with a solution of lithium chloride.

Salt deficiency affecting the excretion of lithium may develop during the situations listed in table 4. Patients with elevated blood pressure often use a low-salt diet. Salt deficiency may also develop during slimming. The amount of food is cut down in order to reduce the intake of calories, but at the same time the amount of salt is reduced, and there may be risk of lithium poisoning unless the patients take extra salt with the diet.

Interaction

Two drugs given simultaneously may show interaction, mutual strengthening or weakening of each other's effects. This may lead to complications and the appearance of side effects, and this possibility should be taken into account when a new drug is prescribed to a patient already taking another drug. This is also true for patients in lithium treatment.

Diuretics (Urine-Producing Drugs, 'Water Pills')

Diuretics are usually employed for treatment of edema, sometimes for treatment of elevated blood pressure, occasionally as part of a slimming cure. Diuretics are widely used drugs. Usually they are fairly innocuous, and instructions for their use just indicate that patients may take the tablets or stop taking the tablets as they like. Taken together with lithium, diuretics are not harmless. They promote the excretion of salt and water, and treatment with diuretics may therefore lead to negative salt and water balance with risk of lithium poisoning. Diuretics should be used only when really needed and under careful control.

Neuroleptics

Lithium is occasionally given together with neuroleptics, particularly haloperidol. The combined administration may lead to increased frequency of side effects, and the use of large doses of neuroleptics can lead to confusion and muscle symptoms. Under appropriate control and when moderate doses of neuroleptics are used, the combination is valuable and without risk.

Antidepressants

If severe depressive recurrences occur during prophylactic lithium treatment, patients should be given antidepressive therapy while at the same time continuing lithium treatment. Lithium and antidepressant drugs are tolerated well together and may even, to some extent, strengthen each other's effects. Occasionally the combination may give rise to increased muscle stiffness, hand tremor, or impaired handwriting, and prolonged administration of antidepressants to patients with previous manias may precipitate new manic episodes. Two newer antidepressants, fluoxetine and fluvoxamine, may not be tolerated well during lithium treatment.

Electric Convulsive Treatment

A depressive relapse during prophylactic lithium treatment may be treated with electric convulsive treatment. In some hospitals lithium administration is stopped temporarily during electroconvulsive treatment.

Other Drugs, the Pill, Alcohol

Caution should be exercised when lithium is given in combination with certain antirheumatic drugs such as phenylbutazone, indomethacin, ketoprofen and diclofenac, and with certain drugs used against high blood pressure, enalapril, captopril, and lisinopril. Lithium may prolong the effect of drugs which block the transfer of signals from nerve to muscle, and this may play a role during electric convulsive treatment and narcosis.

Animal experiments have revealed interaction between lithium and such drugs as morphine, codeine, and amphetamine. This has led to proposals about using lithium for the treatment of drug abuse, but practical experiences have not been encouraging.

There does not seem to be interaction between lithium and sleeping drugs, medicine for anxiety, pain-relieving drugs, cough or cold medications, vitamins, or birth control pills. Nor does lithium treatment appear to influence or be influenced by drugs against epilepsy, thrombosis, or diabetes. Lithium does not change the effects of alcohol.

Caffeine may influence lithium excretion. A constant coffee intake, whether high or low, is of little importance, but change from a high to a low coffee intake, as for example on discharge from hospital, may lead to a rise of serum lithium and necessitate reduction of the lithium dosage.

Pregnancy, Delivery, and Nursing

Malformations

Lithium is frequently given to women in the fertile age range, and the question of possible harm to the unborn child (teratogenic effect) is therefore important. Registration of children born of mothers who were given lithium during the pregnancy has shown a somewhat increased frequency of malformations in the heart and vessels. These findings may, however, exaggerate the risk, since malformed babies are more likely to be reported than normal ones, and a recent prospective study did not show any harmful effects of the treatment. Women, especially those who before lithium treatment had frequent manic or depressive episodes, may therefore continue lithium treatment during the pregnancy; for safety's sake, the child's heart should be examined through fetal echocardiography.

It is not known whether the fetus may be at risk if the father is in lithium treatment at the time of conception.

The Children's Later Development

Most lithium children are born without malformations, but it seemed conceivable that they might reveal developmental abnormalities later. An investigation was therefore carried out of all Scandinavian lithium children who were born without malformations and who had reached the age of 5 years or older. Their mental and physical development was compared with that of their sibs. The study did not reveal any difference between the two groups.

The Effect of Pregnancy on the Treatment

During the last months of pregnancy lithium is excreted more rapidly through the kidneys, and at the time of delivery the excretion rate falls abruptly to the normal. Serum lithium should therefore be tested at relatively short intervals and lithium doses adjusted accordingly. It is advisable to stop lithium treatment a few weeks before delivery and restart it soon after.

Breast-Feeding during Lithium Treatment

Small amounts of lithium pass from the mother's blood into the milk and hence to the nursing child. I have therefore in previous editions of this book advised women in lithium treatment to bottle-feed their children. However, more and more studies indicate that breastfeeding plays an important role for both mother and child, mentally and physically, and it is an open question whether there are more minuses or more plusses in abstaining from breastfeeding during lithium treatment.

Do's and Don'ts in Lithium Treatment

During lithium treatment tablets must be taken regularly each day, even when no signs of disease are present. If the treatment is stopped or the tablet intake neglected, there is risk that the manic and depressive episodes return.

If recurrences of mania or depression develop in spite of lithium treatment, the doctor should be consulted. It may be necessary to increase the dosage or to give supplementary treatment for a time.

Lithium is taken in one or two daily doses, for example morning and evening. The tablets should be washed down with ample amounts of fluid. If patients have difficulty taking tablets with water, they may take them with yoghurt.

If a tablet intake has been forgotten, the patient should not try to make up for it by taking more tablets the next time.

Containers of clear plastic with separate compartments for each day of the week may be used as an aid to remember the regular tablet intake.

Lithium treatment is monitored through laboratory examination of blood samples. The last lithium dose should be taken 12 hours (11–13 hours) before the blood sample is drawn.

Blood samples are drawn once a week during the first weeks, after that at longer intervals according to the doctor's instructions.

The lithium dosage varies from one patient to the other. Dosage adjustment is based on the lithium concentration in the blood serum and the patient's response to the treatment.

Early side effects may occur during the first 1–2 weeks after start of treatment: nausea, stomach ache, loose stools, and fatigue in arms and legs. These side effects usually disappear during continued treatment.

Possible later side effects are: hand tremor, goiter (swelling of the neck due to enlargement of the thyroid gland), myxedema (lowered metabolism due to decreased function of the thyroid gland), polyuria (increased urine production with frequent urination), polydipsia (thirst with increased fluid intake), weight gain, pimples, psoriasis, edema (swelling due to accumulation of water in tissues), and some effect on mental functions. Side effects should be discussed with the doctor, who may be able to reduce or remove them.

During water deficiency (dehydration) and sodium deficiency (salt deficiency) and when lithium is combined with certain other drugs, there is increased risk of lithium poisoning. Risk situations are: physical disease with fever, vomiting, diarrhea, prolonged unconsciousness, narcosis and surgery, low salt diet, slimming diet, treatment with diuretic drugs (water pills) and treatment with certain antirheumatic drugs. In risk situations lithium treatment should be monitored with particular care. The patients must consume ample amounts of water and salt. Under certain circumstances fluid must be administered through infusion (slow injection under the skin or in a vein). In risk situations the patients should watch for signs of impending lithium poisoning.

Lithium should be discontinued during physical illness with fever.

Signs of impending lithium poisoning are the following: apathy, sleepiness, lowered ability to concentrate, muscle weakness, heaviness of the limbs, unsteady gait, marked and possibly irregular tremor, tremor of the jaw, slight muscle twitches, indistinct speech, nausea, vomiting, stomach ache, and diarrhea. If one or more of these signs become prominent, the patient must call the doctor. If the doctor cannot be contacted, the lithium treatment should be discontinued temporarily.

10 Epilogue

We have now reached the end of this book, and I hope it was useful. I have given advice based on personal experience, the experiences of others, and present-day knowledge, but I do not claim to have presented the only or the final truth about manic-depressive illness and about lithium treatment. Others may hold different views and use different procedures, and the acquisition of new knowledge may lead to revision of evaluations and guidelines.

If readers have found things to criticize or if they have suggestions about changes for a possible next edition of the book, I would appreciate being notified. My address is:

The Psychiatric Hospital
Skovagervej 2
DK–8240 Risskov (Denmark)

Supplementary Reading

Goodwin FK, Jamison KR: Manic-Depressive Illness. Oxford, Oxford University Press, 1990.

Jefferson JW, Greist JH, Ackermann DL, Carroll JA: Lithium Encyclopedia for Clinical Practice, ed 2. Washington, American Psychiatric Press, 1987.

Johnson FN: The History of Lithium Therapy. London, MacMillan, 1984.

Johnson FN (ed): Depression and Mania: Modern Lithium Therapy. Oxford, IRL Press, 1987.

Schou M: No help from lithium? About patients who might have been but were not helped by prophylactic lithium treatment. Compr Psychiat 1988;29:83–90.

Schou M: Comments on lithium treatment. Irish J Psychol Med 1991;8:160–167.

Subject Index